D1260371

GOOD GROOMING FOR BOYS

Good Grooming

FOR BOYS

♂

by Rubie Saunders

illustrations by Anne Canevari Green

Franklin Watts
New York / London / Toronto / Sydney / 1989

Revised Edition

Library of Congress Cataloging-in-Publication Data

Saunders, Rubie.
Good grooming for boys / by Rubie Saunders ; illustrated by Anne
Canevari Green.—Rev. ed.
p. cm.
Rev. ed. of: The Franklin Watts concise guide to good grooming for
boys. 1972.
Bibliography: p.
Includes index.
Summary: Advice on cleanliness, diet, exercise, clothes, manners,
and other aspects of personal grooming and behavior.
ISBN 0-531-10768-X
1. Grooming for boys—Juvenile literature. [1. Grooming.]
I. Green, Anne Canevari, ill. II. Saunders, Rubie. Franklin Watts
concise guide to good grooming for boys. III. Title.
RA777.2.S27 1989
646.7'044—dc20
89-30962 CIP AC

To my nephews
Rahman and Raheem

Photographs courtesy of:
Photo Researchers: pp. 12 (David M. Grossman),
41 (Barbara Rios), 44 (Thomas S. England),
45 (Joe Munroe), 48 and 70 (Richard Hutchings),
71 (Larry Nicholson), 76 (Roberta Hershenson),
86 (James Lester); Monkmeyer Press Photos:
pp. 17 (Michal Heron), 26 (Lew Merrim), 30,
37 (Renate Hiller), 52 (P. Conklin), 66 and
78 (Renate Hiller), 83 (Mimi Forsyth); Randy
Matusow: pp. 24, 56, 61, 68; USDA: pp. 40, 57.

Contents

♂

GOOD
GROOMING
FOR
BOYS

GROOMING ISN'T JUST FOR HORSES

You're a teenager or almost one, and there are probably a lot of things that worry you, but how you look shouldn't be one of them. It's fairly easy to develop good grooming habits so you can always face the world with confidence, knowing you look your best.

Why is good grooming important? Because everyone looks and feels better when he or she is clean and appropriately dressed. Then, too, cleanliness—a big part of proper grooming—is essential to good health. Once you have an idea of how your body works and how it's changing as you approach manhood, you'll understand why it's important to keep yourself well groomed and physically fit. And the sooner you get into the habit of a regular grooming routine, the easier it will be.

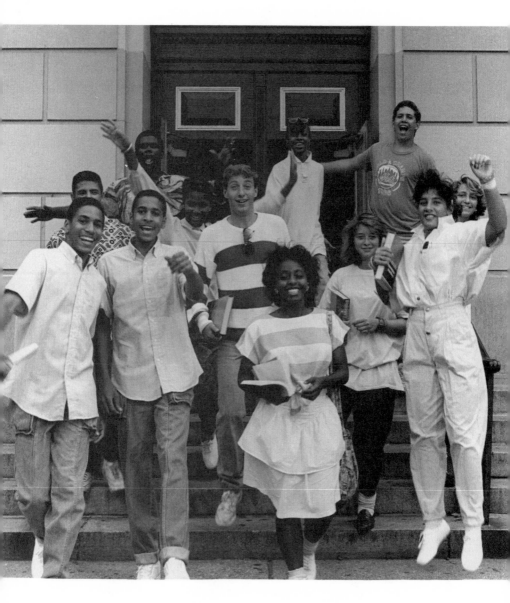

*Being healthy, fit and clean are
the essential parts of good grooming.*

You're never too young to take care of your appearance!

While you should be well groomed for your own sake, you also want to make a good impression on others.

Girls like boys who take pride in their appearance. Parents have one less thing to gripe about when you bathe and change your clothes regularly. Friends prefer being around those who are clean. Sloppiness isn't a sign of masculinity; it's simply the sign of a slob.

When you visit relatives, when you go with a group of friends to a skating rink—whenever you're with people—and you are well groomed, you're saying, "I like you, so I want to look my best for you." That's a good message to convey to anyone. You're also saying, "I like myself," and that, too, makes a good impression on others.

Some boys rebel at the idea of being well groomed because they think it means dressing formally all the time. That is emphatically not true. Look at the men you admire; they don't wear navy blue suits and white shirts all the time. Today's clothes for men are as colorful and as exciting as women's clothes, and there is a great deal of freedom of choice when you shop. Actually, you can dress pretty much as you please and still be well groomed.

FACE
FACTS

Generally the first thing people see when they look closely at you is your face, and certainly that's the part of your body that you are most concerned with. Your face, of course, is covered with skin, and that's what you have to take care of.

The skin on your face, and all over your body, is made up of two layers. The epidermis, the outer layer, is itself made up of outer layers of dead cells that are constantly shedding, and inner layers of live cells. The dermis, the under layer, contains blood capillaries, nerve endings, sweat glands, hair follicles and sebaceous (oil) glands. There are also pores—tiny holes—through both layers of your skin. The epidermis also has cells that produce melanin and carotene, the pigments that give your skin its color. The more melanin you have, the darker your skin will be. Carotene is a yellowish

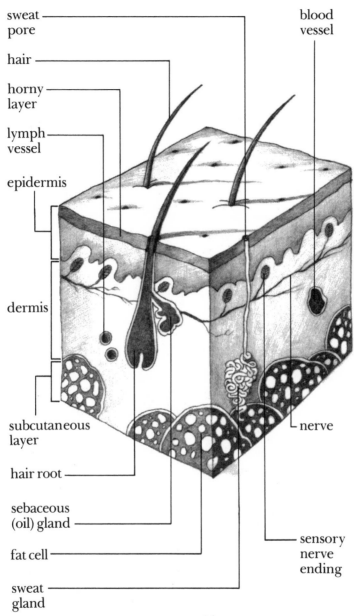

sweat pore

hair

horny layer

lymph vessel

epidermis

dermis

subcutaneous layer

hair root

sebaceous (oil) gland

fat cell

sweat gland

blood vessel

nerve

sensory nerve ending

Human Skin

pigment and is more abundant in some Asian groups.

But whatever color your skin is, whether you're white or black, Native American, Asian or Hispanic, skin is skin and its proper care is the same for everyone. The pigments that determine the color of your skin have no effect on its texture: people of any skin color may have acne or dry skin; blacks need protection from the sun just as much as whites do.

Proper skin care begins with washing your face thoroughly every morning, every night and, if possible, once more during the day. Certainly you should also give your face a good washing after strenuous exercise, and that includes mowing the lawn as well as doing push-ups.

While you've been washing your face since you were a toddler, it's a good idea to review the process. Start by washing your hands; you can't get your face clean with dirty hands. Splash warm water from your hairline to your throat to your ears; use your hands or a soft washcloth for this. Apply soap to the cloth or to your palms and massage it in thoroughly; you want to get rid of those dead skin cells as well as dirt and oil. Massaging in the soap cleans the surface and also helps to remove ground-in dirt that might clog your pores. Rubbing the face briskly also invigorates the skin.

Now rinse the soap completely away; this is as important as removing the dirt because soap left on the skin can dry it too much. Pat your face dry with a clean towel and you're finished.

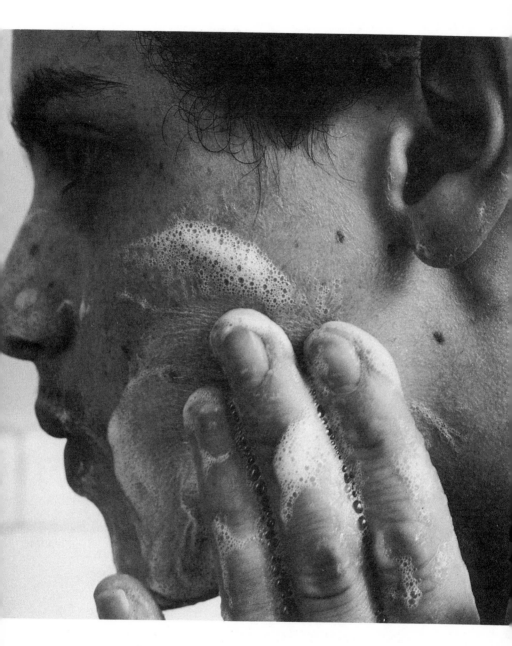

Skin care starts with soap and water.

What kind of soap should you use? Any face soap will do, but if you have an acne problem you can try a medicated soap. Avoid bath soaps, especially those that contain deodorants, because they can overdry the skin.

It's unfortunate, but just when most boys seriously begin to consider their appearance, their faces often break out in acne pimples. The only comforting thing to say about acne is that almost everyone has it; about 98 percent of males and females between the ages of about ten to twenty-four or so have acne to some degree. Mild cases can usually be treated effectively with over-the-counter products that help to dry up excess oil and retard infection; serious acne cases need professional care from doctors who specialize in skin disorders (dermatologists).

What causes acne? It's not your diet, although what you do or don't eat does have an effect on the condition of your skin. Nor is acne caused by dirty skin, but obviously the cleaner your skin is the less susceptible to infection it will be. As you approach puberty, the sebaceous glands in the skin become very active. They produce more oil than ever and produce it faster than it can be eliminated through the pores. The pores become clogged and infection sets in. The result is acne, those pimples that appear usually on your face but can also pop out on your back and, in fact, all over your body.

When you have acne, it's especially important to wash your face three or four times a day. This

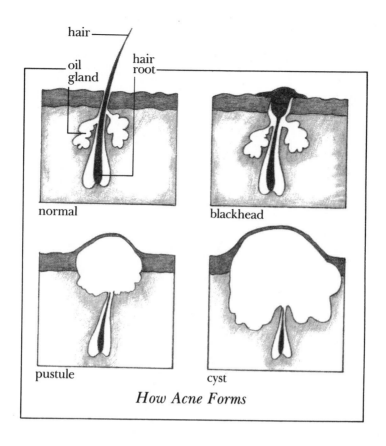

hair

oil gland

hair root

normal

blackhead

pustule

cyst

How Acne Forms

helps to get rid of excess oil and to keep your pores clear, making it harder for infection to set in. While washing alone won't cure acne, it can help to keep it from spreading. Make sure your hands, washcloth and towel are clean. Acne isn't contagious, but it can spread from one part of the body to another.

If your skin feels too tight after washing, and looks dry and flaky, you might be overdrying it. Switch to a milder soap, be careful not to scrub too hard, and cut back to two or three washings a day.

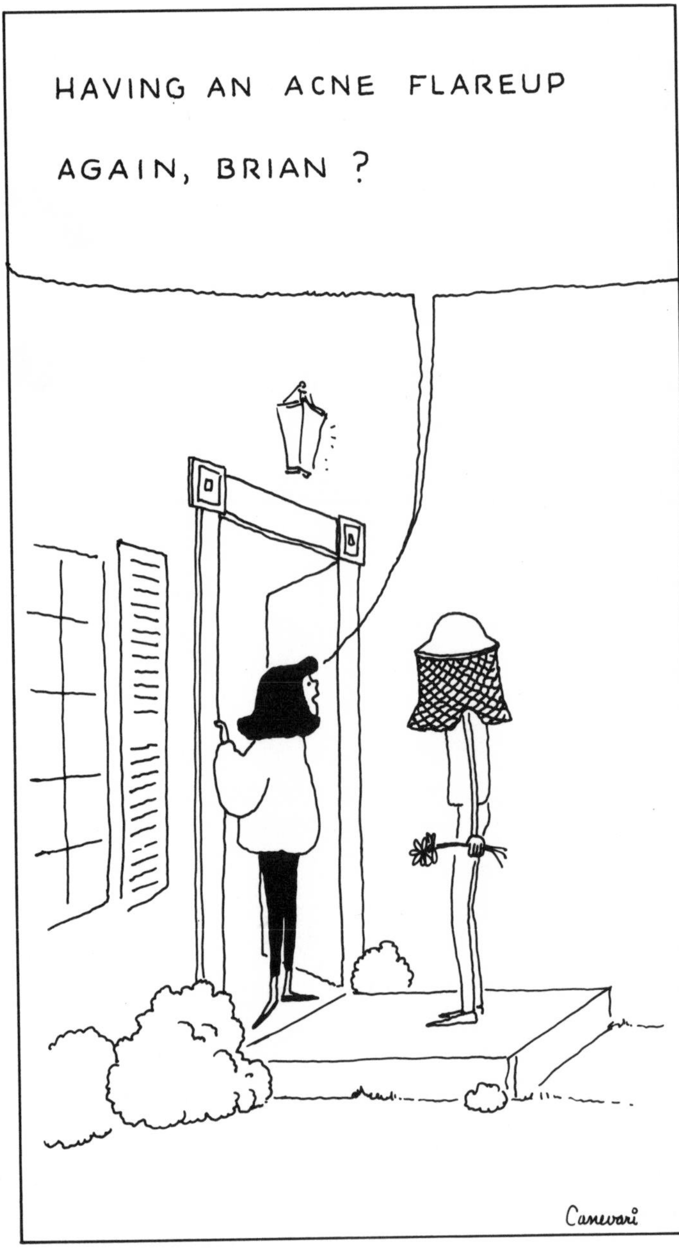
HAVING AN ACNE FLAREUP AGAIN, BRIAN ?
Canevari

Never squeeze acne pimples; that tends to spread the infection, and can also lead to permanent scars. Keep your hands off pimples except when washing and applying medication. Even if you don't have a severe case of acne, it's a good idea to check with the doctor at this point in your life; he or she can tell you the best way to deal with skin problems.

In the recent past, it was thought that foods high in fat caused acne; now it's known that isn't true. However, since your body is producing more oil than ever before, it's a good idea to limit your intake of fatty foods such as chocolate, whole milk, ice cream, potato chips and most other snacks, fried potatoes and fried meats. Your complexion will be better if you eat plenty of leafy vegetables and fresh fruit and drink lots of water and fruit juices.

There are several effective preparations on the market that will help to control acne. Those that dry up excess oil or are medicated to combat infection are best. Most of them are vanishing creams that are absorbed into the skin, so they won't leave your face looking greasy. You can use them during the day as well as at night. There are also astringents—alcohol-containing lotions that you can apply after washing your face to remove excess oil from the skin's surface. There is medical help for severe acne cases; antibiotics and other medications can prevent years of ulcerating cysts. You should definitely see a doctor if you have more than a few acne pimples.

THE
BASICS OF
BATHING

Of course you have more skin than what's on your face; it's all over. Skin, the largest organ in the body, does many other things besides keeping your insides from showing. Skin helps to regulate body temperature and is the means through which the body gets rid of a lot of waste material. You also breathe through your skin; if the body is covered with a nonporous substance, a person can suffocate even if the mouth and nose are uncovered. So it is easy to understand why keeping your skin clean from head to toe is vital to good health.

Actually, good grooming begins with cleanliness. You have to start with a clean body or, no matter what you wear, you won't be really well groomed. If you prefer a shower to a bath, fine; the choice is yours. But whichever you prefer—

and there's no reason why you can't take a bath sometimes and a shower at other times—you have to give yourself a good scrubbing every day.

Daily bathing is a must because you perspire every day, winter as well as summer. And perspiration, which contains oil, allows dirt to cling to your skin. Perspiration also has an odor of its own which tends to become stronger as you grow into your teens. Daily bathing is a matter of cleanliness, a matter of health and a practical matter of living in society.

A bath or shower doesn't have to take a lot of time; about eight to ten minutes should do the job. Surely it's worth ten minutes a day to keep you looking and feeling good!

The time you take bathing will be spent more efficiently if you have the necessary equipment handy. In addition to soap and a washcloth or sponge, it's a good idea to have a nail brush, too. It's great for getting that ground-in dirt from under your fingernails and toenails, and it's also good for elbows, knees and feet. A long-handled brush makes washing your back very easy. If you're going to wash your hair while you bathe, have your shampoo within reach. Fortunately, almost all shampoos are now available in plastic bottles; glass was a hazard when combined with soapy hands and hard bathroom surfaces.

Unless you have a skin problem, any bath soap is fine, but remember that deodorant soaps can dry the skin all over as well as on your face. If

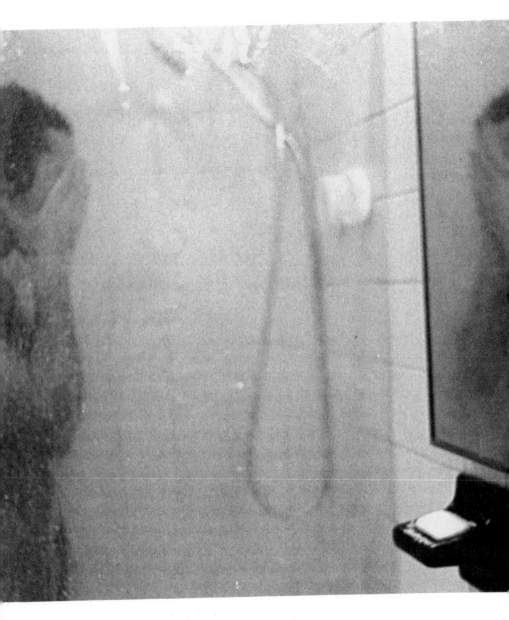

You need a good scrubbing every day.

your skin feels dry and itchy after using a deodorant soap, change to a face soap. It can get you just as clean without irritating your skin.

Now that you have all your supplies within reach, you're ready to step into the shower or tub. Use water that's comfortably warm; test it with your hand or toe first. Start by washing your face as described in "Face Facts." Now soap up your washcloth or sponge and scrub your neck, both front and back. Don't forget your ears; your little finger, with the cloth wrapped around it, will do a good job here inside and out.

The simplest way to get your back clean, next to asking someone to scrub it for you, is with a long-handled back brush. But you can also do a good job with a washcloth. Hold one corner of the washcloth in one hand with the opposite corner in the other. With one hand over your shoulder and the other behind your back, use a back-and-forth and up-and-down motion to cover the whole area.

Use the cloth or sponge to wash your genitals thoroughly. This is particularly important, for health as well as for cleanliness.

Wash your arms, from shoulder to fingernails, and don't forget to use the nail brush on your elbows and knuckles. Do the same with your legs and feet. Rinse the soap off completely; then towel yourself dry, rubbing briskly. Now you can step out of the bathroom ready to face the world—once you put on some clothes!

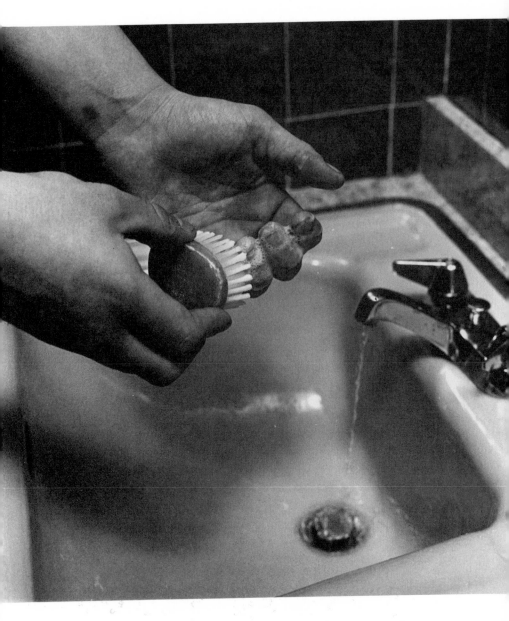

*A nail brush is useful for scrubbing
nails, knuckles and elbows.*

If you follow this routine every day, using the same procedure whether you sit in a tub of water or stand under a shower, you'll discover that getting yourself clean is a pleasant experience. While it should take you only about ten minutes, plus an additional five if you shampoo your hair, you will find that lying back in a tub filled with warm water is a great way to relax tired muscles. And standing under a shower invigorates as well as cleans you. Tub or shower, bathing can refresh your mind as well as your body, so don't neglect it.

Should you shower in the morning or at night? The choice is up to you. In the winter, it might be more comfortable for you to do it at night, while in the summer you might prefer the morning. Actually, it doesn't matter when you shower as long as you make sure you give your body a thorough cleaning every day.

ARE DEODORANTS FOR YOU?

If you watch television or read magazines and newspapers, you are certainly aware of deodorants. While most of the advertisements are directed at adults, everybody, from about the age of ten, needs more protection than a daily shower can provide. This is especially true during the early teens when body chemistry changes as you develop adult characteristics.

Deodorants are available in various forms—roll-ons, solids, creams, powders and soaps. There are plain deodorants (although they are not too common these days) and those that are antiperspirants as well. Whichever you use is a matter of personal preference, but for the sake of those with whom you come into contact, please use something! Even if you shower with a deodorant soap, chances are you need additional protection.

The difference between a plain deodorant and one that's also an antiperspirant is simple. The first eliminates the odor of perspiration; the second stops the perspiration itself (or most of it). Both are used under the arms and should be applied immediately after bathing. Putting any type of deodorant on unclean skin defeats its purpose.

In general, boys nine or ten don't have a real problem with perspiration; its odor is very faint. But as you near your teens, the body changes. You not only perspire more, but your perspiration also has a much stronger odor. You can shower at seven in the morning and by noon, if you haven't used an effective deodorant, people near you can smell your perspiration.

A few people still think that strong perspiration odors are manly, but if you've ever sat next to a boy in school or on a bus who smelled, you know it's unpleasant. Deodorants aren't just for girls; boys need them, too. Buy small sizes of deodorants until you find one that works effectively for you. Then you can invest in the larger, more economical sizes. It doesn't matter if you choose a roll-on, solid or cream; they all work equally well. Deodorant powders can be applied all over the body; they are usually used in combination with an underarm deodorant.

Your underarms aren't the only places where odors can develop. Because they're encased in shoes of one sort or another most of the time, feet can smell unpleasant, too. Pay careful attention to your feet when bathing; make sure you wash between

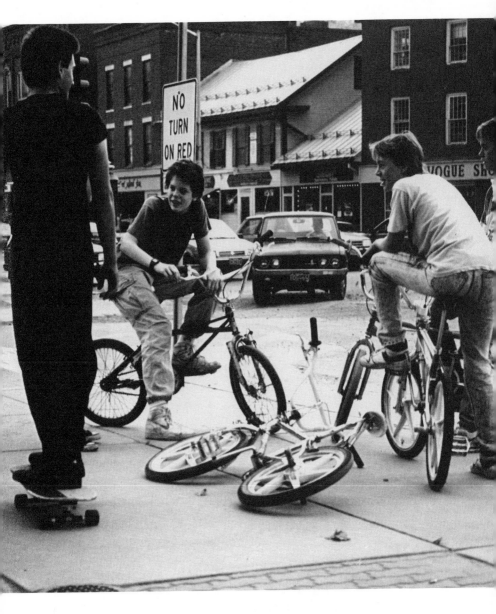

*Active, healthy teens need a deodorant
along with a daily scrubbing.*

each toe. Applying a deodorant powder to your feet—rub it in well, don't just sprinkle it on—after washing and drying them will eliminate bad foot odors. Also sprinkle powder in your sneakers to keep them odor-free.

If you have athlete's foot—a very itchy infection between the toes—you can buy medications to combat it. Some are liquid, some are creams, some are powders. Using a medicated powder on your feet and in all your shoes and sneakers will combat the fungus that causes athlete's foot.

YOU ARE
WHAT
YOU EAT

Your diet—the foods you eat every day—has a great deal to do with the condition of your skin and hair as well as with your general health. The healthier your diet, the better you look and feel. Whether you think you're overweight, underweight or just right, you still need three well-balanced meals a day.

You've already learned that fatty foods aren't particularly good for your complexion; they're also not good for your general health. Eating large amounts of food high in fats and cholesterol, such as whole milk, butter, ice cream, chocolate and fatty meats, may lead to serious health problems in the future. The cholesterol causes deposits to build up on the walls of your arteries, reducing the space through which blood can flow. This can increase the risk of heart attacks, strokes and other serious illnesses. Reducing your intake of high-cholesterol foods now can prolong your life, so eat smart!

While some salt is important for good health, most Americans consume far too much salt. Large amounts of salt may contribute to hypertension, or high blood pressure. You should reduce the amount of salt you eat. If you use a little less each day, your taste buds will learn to do without a lot of salt. One fringe benefit of a low-salt diet is that you learn what food actually tastes like. You can season food with lemon juice, pepper and other spices and herbs instead of burying the flavor with spoonfuls of salt.

You need to be sure your diet includes good sources of proteins, vitamins and minerals. You also need high-fiber foods such as leafy vegetables, bran cereals and whole-grain or multigrain breads and cereals. Eating these foods regularly may reduce the risks of developing certain kinds of cancer.

If you think a healthy diet is a dull one, you're wrong. You can eat a wide variety of foods, prepared in many different ways, and still have well-balanced meals. For example, a dinner that consists of a broiled lamb chop (remove most of the fat before cooking), a baked potato with no-cholestrol margarine and chives, and broccoli spears is as tasty as it is healthy. Add whole-grain rolls or bread, skim or low-fat milk and fresh fruit for dessert and you have a satisfying meal.

Eating healthy doesn't mean you can never have ice cream or cake or pie; nor do you have to

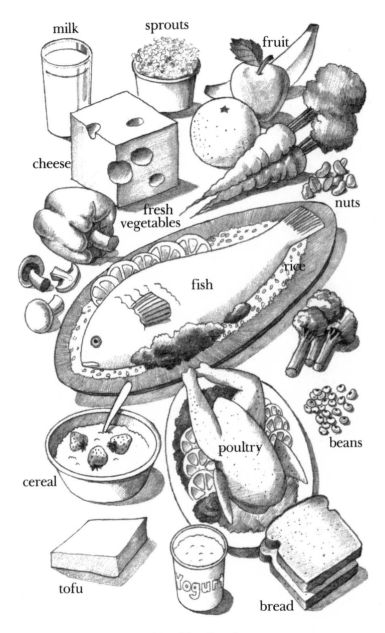

milk

sprouts

fruit

cheese

fresh
vegetables

nuts

rice

fish

beans

poultry

cereal

tofu

bread

Healthy Food

give up hamburgers and french fries. It simply means that you should limit the number of times you eat such foods. Let's face it, you don't have to stop at a fast-food place every day after school. And it probably won't be hard to convince Mom and Dad that broiling, baking or roasting meat, fish and poultry is better than frying. You can enjoy a steak for dinner on Tuesday, but have fish or chicken (preferably the breast with the skin removed) or stir-fried vegetables the next day.

Do the family a favor and buy a cookbook that has recipes for dishes that are good for the entire family. Such foods may require less preparation time than meals that are high in fats and low in fiber! The chef in your household will certainly be impressed with your good sense and your concern for the whole family's well-being. Remember Mom and Dad need to eat right just as much as you and your kid sister do.

Weighing too much or too little is a problem for boys as well as girls. You can forget about an "ideal" weight because there's no such thing. Most weight charts are meaningless because they usually consider only age and height in determining what a person should weigh. Other factors also influence your optimum weight, so that you look and feel your best.

Take a look at the boys in your class. Several of them may be the same height, but each of them can have a different skeletal structure. A boy who is about five feet (1.5 m) tall with large bones will naturally weigh quite a bit more than a boy of the same height with small bones. And a boy who is very active probably will weigh less than his friend who spends most of his free time in front of a television set even if they're both the same height and have the same skeletal structure.

If you have any questions about your own weight, check with your doctor. He or she will consider your age, height, skeletal structure and how active or inactive you are and tell you what you should weigh.

Contrary to what you may have heard, most overweight people, young and old, simply eat too much and don't exercise enough. Often they don't eat well-balanced meals, either. Even though you are probably not the one who decides what's served for dinner, you can do a lot on your own to shed any unwanted pounds.

The first step in losing weight is to eliminate between-meal snacks. That's easier said than done because you probably feel hungry all the time. But french fries, potato chips and candy bars are not only too oily for your complexion, they're also high in calories and fairly low in nutrition. If you eat three well-balanced meals a day, it isn't really necessary to raid the refrigerator each time you pass it. Your body will soon become accustomed to having less food so those gnawing hunger pangs will disappear.

It will be easier to avoid a midmorning snack, which too often is a candy bar, if you eat a good breakfast. Quickly swallowing a glass of juice and munching on a piece of toast as you dash out the

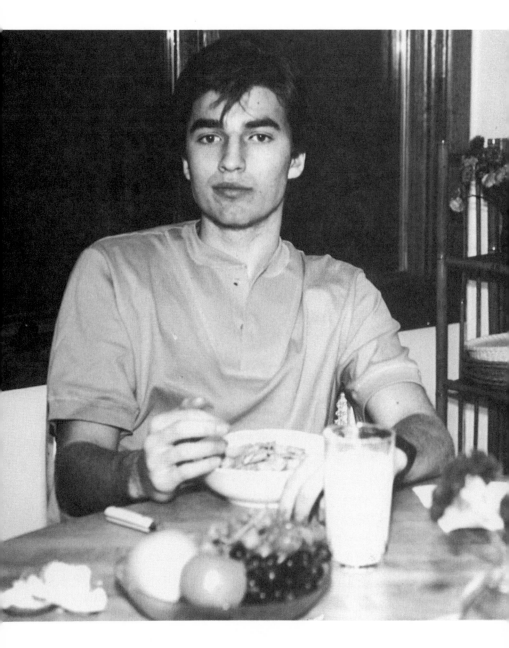

A healthy breakfast starts a good diet.

door hardly provides you with enough energy to last until lunch. And whether you want to lose weight or gain it, a good breakfast is a must.

One way to start the day right is to vary what you eat. Cold cereals can be a bore after a while, so have eggs or pancakes or cottage cheese with fruit once a week. No time for an elaborate meal in the morning's mad rush to get to school on time? Then put a large glass of skim or low-fat milk into the blender, add three drops of vanilla or almond extract or a ripe banana, strawberries or other fruit. Blend at the highest speed for thirty seconds and—presto!—you have a good breakfast you can drink. A slice of whole-wheat toast, with a fruit spread, or a muffin completes your meal-on-the-run.

Or make a breakfast sandwich using whole-grain bread or rolls, bagels or pita bread and grilled cheese or your favorite filling. Just make sure it's low in salt.

Actually, you can eat whatever you please for breakfast as long as the meal includes bread, fruit, and milk, cheese, meat, eggs or another protein source. There's no reason why you can't have a chop from last night's dinner if you feel like it!

You can understand the importance of a good breakfast if you count the hours between yesterday's dinner and today's lunch. That's a long time to go without eating a real meal. It could cause you trouble in your morning classes. If you have gym in the morning, for example, you might miss more baskets than you make. It's worth getting up a little earlier in the morning so you'll have time for a good breakfast.

If possible, have a hot meal at lunch. If the food in your school cafeteria isn't to your liking, a Thermos bottle filled with your favorite soup, with a sandwich and fruit for dessert, will provide you with a nourishing meal in the middle of the day. However, most schools make an effort to provide lunches that are both tasty and nutritious. The United States government has established guidelines for school lunches that include such foods as pizza, hamburgers and even hot dogs, so check what your cafeteria offers.

Remember that you can eat a heavy meal at lunch without adding pounds if you balance it with a lighter dinner. Since practically everyone is more active between lunch and dinner than between dinner and bedtime, you can see how it's possible to burn up those midday calories.

After school, eat fresh fruit or raw vegetables instead of foods higher in calories and lower in nutrition such as sodas and cake. If you and your friends usually stop after school for a snack, have fruit juice instead of a carbonated soda.

At dinner, eat lots of steamed vegetables with lemon juice instead of salt; a modest portion of meat, fish, a tofu dish or poultry, and a small serving of starches—potatoes, rice or pasta. A casserole that contains dried beans, grains and leafy vegetables is a good base for a nutritious meal. Don't cut out starches entirely; you need the nutrients they contain for proper growth. If you are practically starving at bedtime, have more fruit or fruit juice.

You can also lose some weight just by reduc-

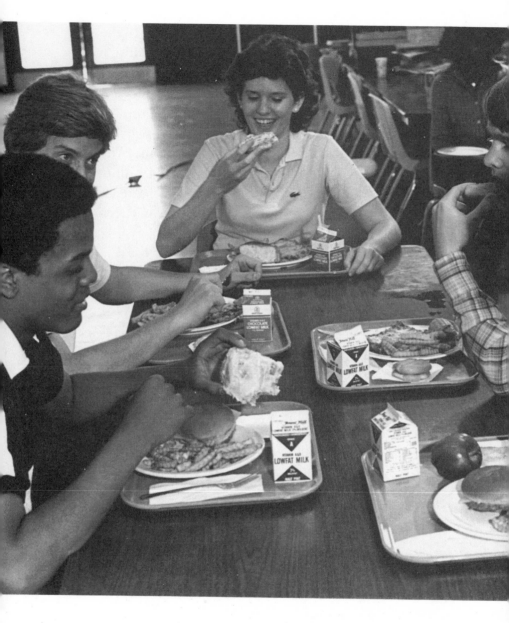

School cafeterias offer choices so you can find the kind of lunch you need.

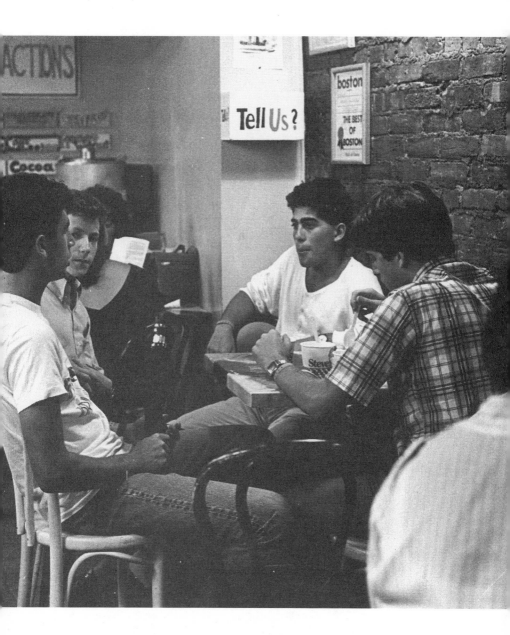

An after-school snack can be orange juice
or ice cream—the choice is yours.

ing the amount of salt you eat. The more salt you ingest, the more fluid the body retains, and water weighs a lot! When you cut down on salt, you will find that you have to go to the bathroom more often; that's okay.

Once you follow a routine of eating smaller portions of three good meals a day—going easy on the starches but not eliminating them completely—you will lose weight. The only foods you have to avoid are the snacks that are high in calories, salt, fats and cholesterol and low in nutrition. But because you're still growing, you can't go on the crash diets you might find in magazines and newspapers without risking your health; actually, no one at any age can.

You might be uncomfortable the first couple of days of your diet because you feel hungry all the time. Be patient; that will pass as your system becomes accustomed to less food. You'll also notice that you might take off two pounds (.9 k) almost immediately, then there will be no weight loss for a week or more. Relax; there's nothing wrong with your scale or with you, it's just that you've hit a plateau. One morning you'll step on the scale and it will look as if you've lost five pounds (2.25 k) overnight. You really haven't lost it that fast; it's just been coming off gradually all the while.

To have an accurate record of your weight, you should weigh yourself at approximately the same time of day because your weight fluctuates during the day. First thing in the morning is a good time; you'll probably weigh less then than you do before bedtime.

In addition to watching what you eat, exercise is vitally important to any weight-reduction program. Walking briskly, riding a bike, running, skating, or team sports are good ways to keep trim. If you're not athletic, walk to the library instead of asking someone to drive you. If you move at a good pace, not merely dragging yourself along, you'll use muscles that certainly need exercising. Not only will you look better, you'll feel better, too.

If you want to gain weight, you can have some high-calorie snacks—more than your friend who wants to lose weight. Remember that nutrition is important for you, too, and you still want to limit the fats you eat. You can increase the number of calories in your diet by choosing foods high in proteins and carbohydrates. Eating two apples is a better idea than eating a candy bar!

If you don't have much of an appetite, you can add weight by having four meals a day. The extra meal is your after-school snack. Have a sandwich along with milk or an ice cream soda. For a bedtime snack, have a bowl of cereal or a muffin and a glass of milk. By eating four meals a day instead of three, you'll find it easier to consume more food during a twenty-four-hour period. Nothing is worse for someone with a poor appetite than being faced with a plate piled high with food. That's why it's a good idea to add an extra meal to your daily menu.

Your appetite will also improve if you make a point of getting some outdoor exercise every day. Try walking home from school instead of taking

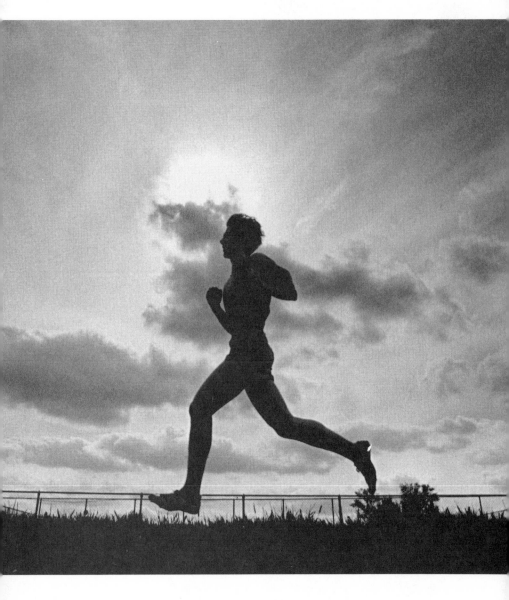

Exercising for health and fitness
is a part of grooming.
And exercise is fun, too.

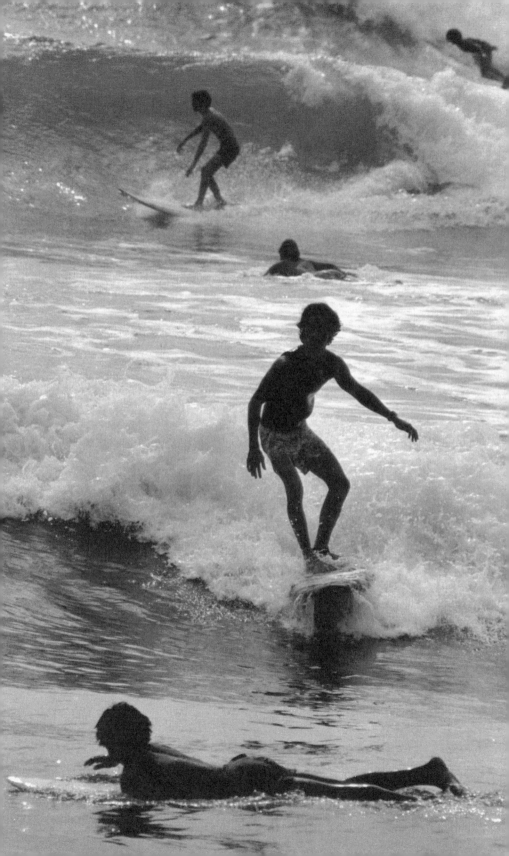

the bus, or jog with friends regularly. Even if sports don't appeal to you, play a game of catch with a friend. You can't expect to gain weight if you sit around all day and only nibble at your food. Besides, exercise will also tone up any sagging muscles.

Whether you want to gain or lose weight, remember you're still growing. Crash diets aren't for you, nor are meals that are too heavy or too light in starches or those that don't include items from each of the four basic food groups—meat and related foods (poultry, fish, eggs and beans), vegetables and fruits, milk and milk products, and grains (cereals and breads). You also need fiber in your diet, so dig into leafy vegetables and whole-grain cereals and breads. But cut down on fatty meats, eggs, butter and other foods with a high fat and cholesterol content; they aren't good for anyone.

Every member of the family, from your baby brother to your great-grandmother, needs balanced meals, so your parents don't have to cook special things for you. All you have to do is eat more to gain, or less to lose.

STRETCH, BEND, AND PULL

Do you feel tired a lot of the time even though you get enough sleep? That can happen if you don't exercise. Stretching your muscles will improve your appearance, and you'll feel much better, too. Before any exercise—whether it's walking, running, playing basketball or working out in a gym—take a few minutes to stretch and loosen all your muscles, from neck to toes.

Start your exercise program by improving your posture. No matter how clean you are or how well dressed, if your posture is bad you won't look your best. Whether you realize it or not, the way you stand, sit and walk tells a lot about the kind of person you are. Sprawling all over a chair when you sit, slouching when you walk, looking like a pretzel when you stand in line at the school cafeteria—all these indicate poor posture.

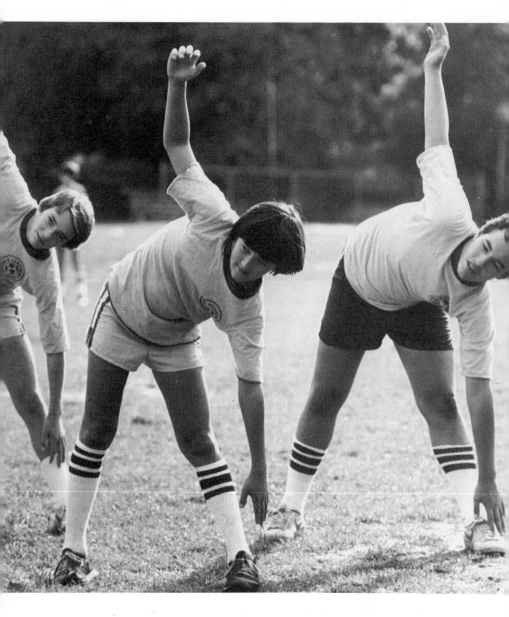

Whether you're going to play soccer, bike or jog, every muscle needs to be stretched first.

Don't think you have to be ramrod-stiff at all times; that's not good posture any more than slouching is. Actually, it's not hard to learn how to stand, sit and walk properly. Once you do, you'll be pleased to discover that many of the problems you may have had with your body will disappear.

Start with good standing posture. Look at yourself in a full-length mirror. Is your head practically buried in your neck? Does your chest have a caved-in look? Is your stomach sticking out? Are your knees bent? If your answer is yes to any of these questions, it's high time you did something constructive about your posture.

Still facing the mirror, imagine that a strong string is attached to the top of your head. Now imagine someone directly above you is slowly pulling that string up to the ceiling. As the string tightens, your head comes out of your neck, your chest expands, your stomach flattens and your knees straighten. That is how you should stand. Your arms should hang loosely at your sides; don't hold them so stiffly you lock your elbows.

Here is a simple exercise to help you achieve and maintain good standing posture. Stand with your back to a wall and your heels about a hand's length away from the base of the wall. Your back and shoulders should touch it. With your hands straight at your sides, but not rigid, and your head and shoulders back, bend your knees and, very slowly, slide down the wall until your butt touches the floor. Hold that position for a slow count of five, then push your body up the wall without us-

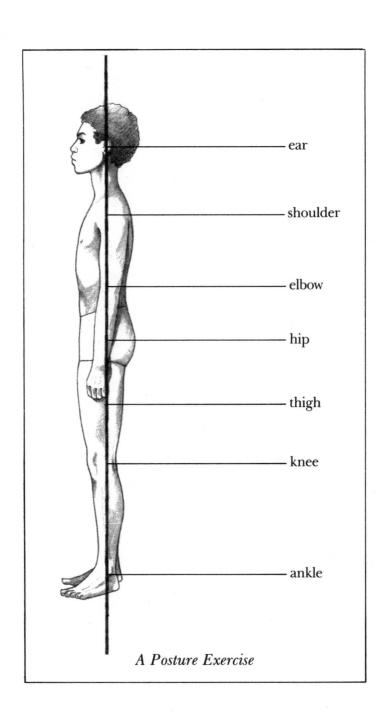

ear

shoulder

elbow

hip

thigh

knee

ankle

A Posture Exercise

ing your hands. As you move up, tense your buttocks, keep your hips tucked under and press the small of your back to the wall. Do this up-and-down-the-wall exercise about four times the first day; add another each succeeding day until you can comfortably do ten a day.

Another way to check your posture is to hang a piece of string, longer than you are tall, with a weight at the bottom end, in front of a full-length mirror. Stand sideways with your hands at your sides. If you are standing correctly, the string should cut across your ear, shoulder, elbow, hip, thigh, knee and ankle. If it doesn't, adjust your stance until it does.

Good posture is more than the way you stand, it also involves sitting and walking. When you sit, your back should be straight and your feet should be flat on the floor. Of course, there are times when you want to relax, perhaps with a book, and there's no reason why you can't. But relaxing doesn't mean sitting on the nape of your neck and the base of your spine with your feet sprawled in front of you. Nor do you have to curl yourself into a knot. You can cross your legs or even sit on one of them if you choose, but don't sit in such a way that you squeeze your insides together!

Remember what you learned about good standing posture and use it when you're walking; don't *schlump* along like an elephant with sore feet. To get the feel of good walking posture, start with your back against the wall. Now walk away from it, but don't push yourself; just step away from

[51]

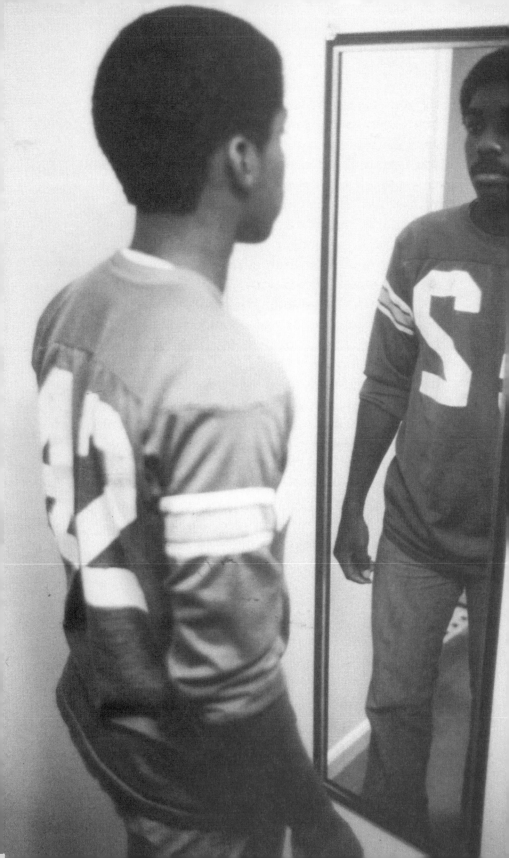

the wall. Don't lead with your head, stomach or hips. Your body should be straight and proud. Imagine there's an arrow painted on the floor as you stroll along. Your heels should be on the shaft; your toes slightly to the left and right of it. Swing your arms; this not only helps to keep your balance, but it's a natural motion when walking.

If you're interested in sports, you know the importance of good coordination. In a way, walking is a kind of sport, and proper posture will help you to develop a well-coordinated walk. It will also help you move around the baseball diamond, the basketball court, the football or soccer field. And did you ever hear of an uncoordinated bowler breaking two hundred?

What other reason is there for developing good posture? Take the example of two boys, Andy and Walter. Both are bright, ambitious and hard-working. There is an opening at a local supermarket for a boy to pack groceries Friday nights and Saturdays, and both Walter and Andy apply for the job. They have to be interviewed by the manager, who will choose only one of them.

Andy slouches into the manager's office, sprawls on the chair and answers questions in a muffled voice. Because of the way he's sitting, he can't get enough air into his lungs to speak properly.

A full-length mirror can
help you check your posture.

[53]

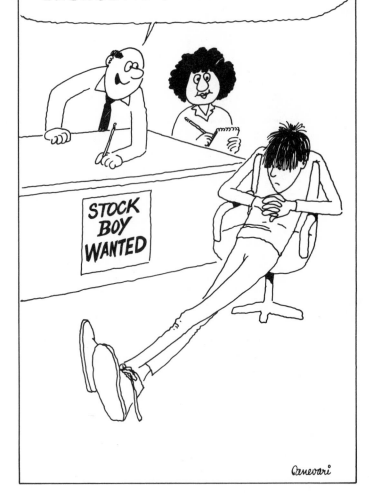

Then Walter comes in, walking tall—erect but not stiff. He sits straight in the chair, his feet flat on the floor. He speaks in a clear voice.

Which boy do you think the manager hired? You're right; he hired Walter. His walking, standing and sitting posture indicated that he was alert and energetic, while Andy gave the impression of being lazy and irresponsible. He really isn't, but in the brief time the interview lasted, how could the manager tell?

With good posture, you give the impression of alertness, vitality and self-confidence. Prospective employers value these traits, and teachers, parents and other boys and girls do, too. So make sure your posture says good things about you. Walk tall!

Walking briskly is the easiest way to exercise; you can do it at your convenience and it doesn't require any special equipment except comfortable shoes or sneakers. It's a great way to tone up your leg muscles and if you squeeze a tennis ball in each hand in rhythm with your pace, you'll also strengthen your arm muscles. Or you can carry an unopened can of soup in each hand; bend your arm at the elbow and bring it up to your shoulder as you step along.

If you haven't done much exercising, start walking briskly for about twenty minutes—ten minutes going and ten minutes coming. Increase the length of your walk gradually to at least an hour. If you can cover four miles (6.4 km) in an

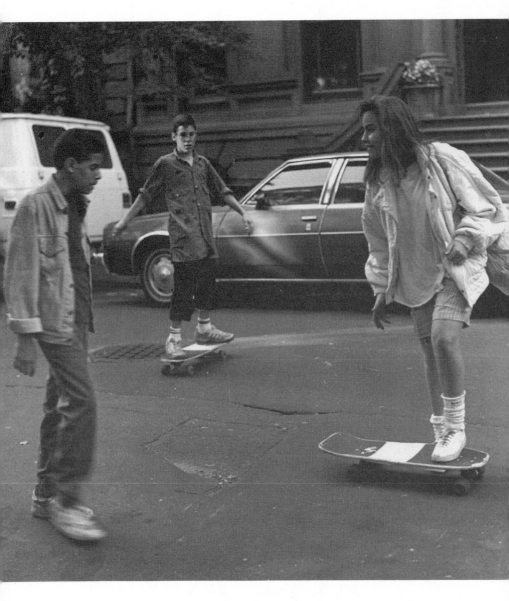

Good posture and coordination are important in walking, playing basketball, or mastering a skateboard.

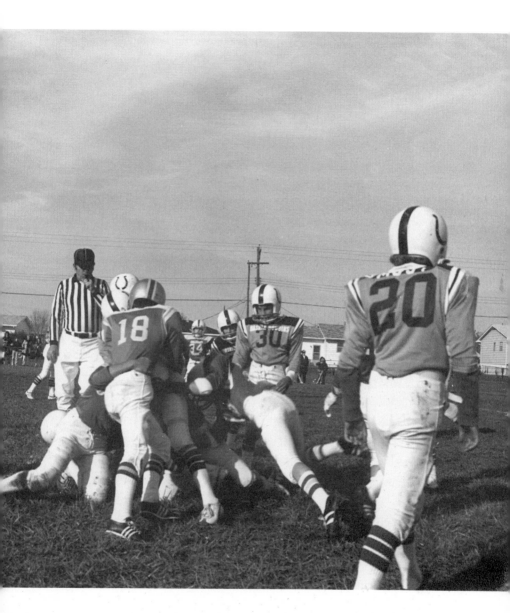

*Football, track, basketball
and other team sports offer
good exercise.*

hour, you're walking at a pace that will improve your muscle tone; it will also increase your lung capacity. Take long strides; you want to feel those thigh muscles stretching.

Push-ups and sit-ups are fine exercises for strengthening your arms and upper body and for tightening your stomach muscles. Do them while you watch television; time yourself by counting commercials (most of them are ten, thirty or sixty seconds each).

But exercising doesn't have to be a solitary effort. Playing soccer with your friends is great for the legs; basketball, tennis and baseball do wonders for your arms; football is good exercise for both arms and legs. And to exercise almost every muscle in your body with a minimum of exertion, swim a couple of laps in a pool.

Running and jogging are also great ways to stretch muscles and to make you feel good both mentally and physically. As with any exercise, start slowly; don't try to run a marathon the first day! And make sure you have the proper footwear; the salesperson at a sporting-goods store can help you find the type of sneaker that is best suited for the kind of running, jogging or walking you want to do.

You need to exercise if you're losing weight, to prevent your muscles from becoming flabby. Exercise is also important if you want to gain weight, as it keeps your muscles toned. But even if your weight isn't a problem, exercise is essential to good health, so get off your butt!

GOOD
NIGHT

Have you ever stayed up late on a school night to watch a television show? Remember how you felt the next day? Getting up in the morning was pure torture, and by one or two o'clock in the afternoon your eyes felt as if they were full of sand and ready to fall out. It was pretty hard for you to understand what the teacher was saying.

An experience like that can teach you the importance of sleep. It is the time your body refreshes and renews itself, and you're cheating yourself if you don't allow as many hours as necessary for sleeping. In every twenty-four-hour period, you must give your body a good rest. Generally, that means eight to ten hours of sleep every night if you want to function properly and look like a human being instead of a zombie. While it's true that some people seem to get along with less sleep, you need to learn what your own body needs rather than copy what your best friend does.

If you feel rested and can cope with school and fun after only seven hours of sleep, fine. But if you practically fade out by midafternoon, you obviously need more sleep at night. Does it make sense to view your world through sleep-filled eyes just for the sake of a television show?

A good night's sleep is important every night. On school nights, make a practice of going to bed seven to ten hours before you have to get up. On other nights it's all right to stay up later because you can sleep later in the morning. During the teens, many boys seem to need close to twelve hours of sleep a night. By the time you're thirty-five or forty, six hours a night might be all you need. But for now, you might need almost twice as many hours of sleep as your father.

To get the most out of the time you spend sleeping, open the window in your bedroom winter and summer. Breathing fresh air as you sleep is very refreshing. Air conditioners and radiators remove moisture from the air, and very dry air can dry the membranes in your nose and mouth. A bowl of water in front of the air conditioner or a pan of water on top of the radiator can restore needed moisture to the air.

With a healthy diet, a fit body and enough sleep, you can do anything.

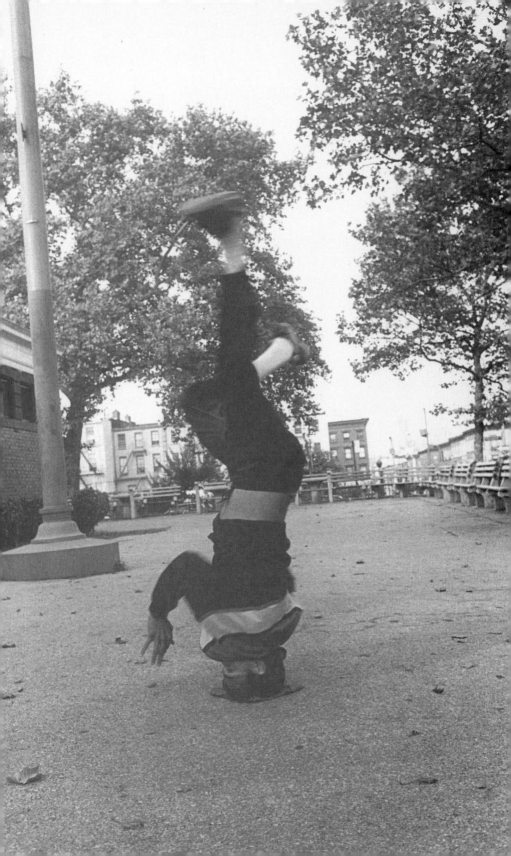

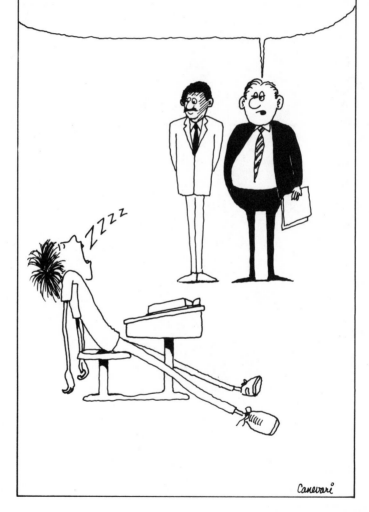

Your mattress should be firm enough to support your body; a soft mattress isn't really as restful. And sleep in pajamas rather than in your underwear; it's more sanitary.

Once in a while you might have trouble falling asleep; worrying about the book report you haven't even started, for example, might keep you wide awake. To overcome this, get into a comfortable position and breathe in deeply, hold it for a count of three, then slowly exhale. Repeat until you are relaxed enough to fall asleep—usually within five or ten minutes. Another trick is to list all fifty states in alphabetical order; concentrating on that will help push your worries out of your mind. You could be sound asleep before you get to Maine!

Sufficient sleep is important for good health, and you'll also look better, do better in school and have more fun during your free time when you get enough rest.

CLOTHES
MAKE
THE
MAN

"Are you going out dressed like *that?*"

How many times have your parents said that to you? If your only answer is, "Heck, all the guys dress like this," remember that you are an individual; you don't have to be a carbon copy of anyone else.

It's natural for you to want to dress like your friends, but you don't have to choose between looking exactly like everybody else and sticking out like a sore thumb. You can dress in style and still be an individual. All you have to do is pick clothes you like that look good on you. Even if you're wearing a sports shirt and jeans just like all the other boys, the style and colors you choose can reflect your own taste.

When it comes to selecting your clothes, you might be faced with a bewildering choice of colors and styles; don't let that scare you. You'll have an easier time choosing the shapes and colors you want to wear if you learn something about how they relate to you.

Take colors first. When it comes to shirts and other items worn fairly close to your face, you have to consider not only whether you like them, but how they look on you. This is easier if you know something about skin tones.

Practically everyone's complexion is either predominantly red-pink, yellow or brown—that's true of Native Americans, black people, Asians, Hispanics and white people. To discover what colors are best for your particular skin tone, hold various shades to your cheek. If at all possible, do this near a window; natural light won't distort the colors the way incandescent or fluorescent lights will. Does bright red make your skin look yellowish? Or does it look rosier? Now hold different shades of blue, one at a time, to your face. What effect do they have on your complexion? Do the same with black and shades of green. You'll be able to see for yourself which colors are good for you and which ones aren't.

Being familiar with this technique will help you make the right choice when it comes to selecting colors. With the almost unlimited range of colors available in shirts and sweaters, you'll have no trouble finding those that are not only in style but just right for you.

Colors can also affect aspects of your appearance other than your skin tone. Are you over-

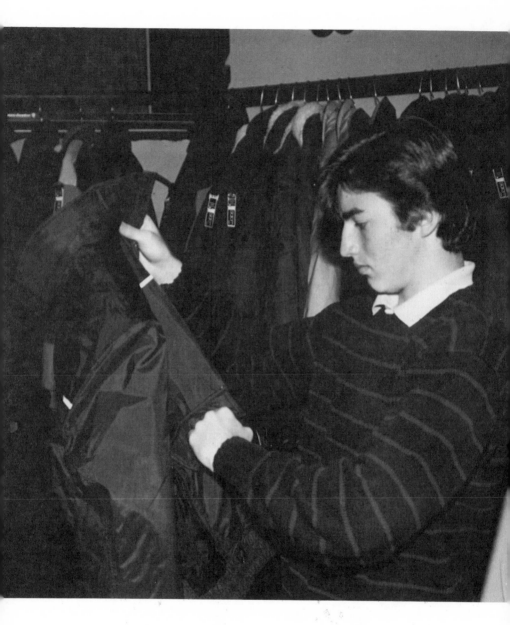

The clothes you choose reflect your taste.

weight? Then pick solid colors rather than splashy prints and large checks. Vertical stripes will make you appear slimmer than horizontal ones, and shirts and pants in the same color will also make any excess pounds less noticeable. While many people think wearing a shirt outside the pants makes a person look slimmer, that isn't true. You'll look thinner with your shirt tucked inside your pants because your waist will show and it will look smaller. Clothes that are too tight draw attention to your weight.

You may think pants are pants, period. But styles in men's pants change as often as the hemlines on women's skirts. One season flared bottoms may be in style; the next season everyone's wearing tapered-leg pants. And six months later the straight leg is in fashion. Cuffs and pleats at the waist are other styles that come and go in men's pants. Flared bottoms look better on thin boys than on those who are overweight, who may find pants with straight legs are a good choice. Whether you're plump or thin, unless your legs are reasonably straight, stay away from tapered-leg pants. They make bowlegs look even more curved.

Once you know how to pick the colors, patterns and shapes that do the most for you, you should also know *what* to wear *when*. Any well-groomed young man realizes that it isn't enough to have clothes that look right on him, he has to dress for each occasion. Even in today's informal world, there is a place for different types of clothes.

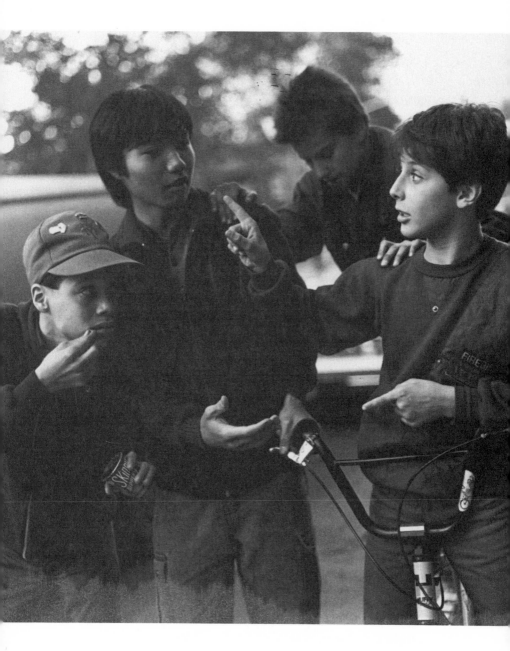

After-school clothes can be comfortable and informal.

For example, your father may prefer brightly colored shirts and suits tailored in the latest fashion, but if he has to go to a funeral he would wear more subdued clothing. In other words, he's dressing for the occasion, and that's what you should do, too.

Torn, grease-stained jeans are fine for playing football with your buddies, but not for school. Going skating with your friends doesn't mean you have to dress up in a shirt and tie, but don't look as if you slept in your clothes.

If you're going to dinner at the home of relatives, it would be thoughtful if you dressed a little more carefully than you would for hanging out with your friends. Of course, what you wear may depend upon your family's customs, but chances are a turtleneck shirt and neat pants would be in keeping with the mental image you have of yourself without offending an elderly aunt and uncle. On some occasions a jacket might be a good idea. When in doubt about what to wear to a family function, ask Mom or Dad what they'd like you to wear. Even if their choice strikes you as impossible, you might go along with it. Probably none of your friends will see you anyway, if that worries you.

Whatever clothes you wear, they should be clean. In these days with a washing machine in practically every house and laundromats on almost every street, there's no excuse for you to wear clothes that are dirty and smelly. Change your underwear and socks every day; there's little point in

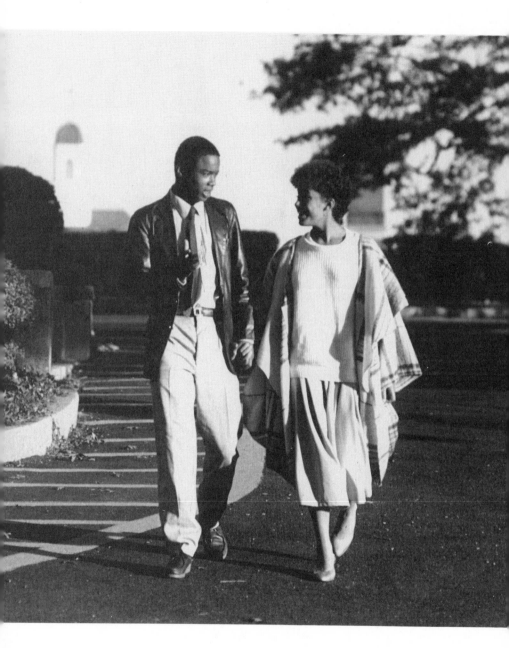

There are times when you need to dress up.

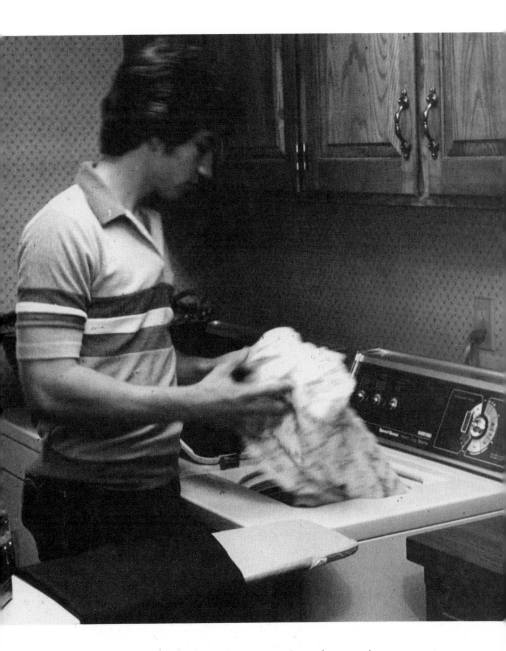

Clean clothes are another part of good grooming.

taking a daily shower if you put on yesterday's underwear. Jackets, suits and pants that have to be dry-cleaned should be checked to see if they need cleaning before you put them on. Better yet, check them after you wear them; you can take them to the cleaners so they'll be ready the next time you want to wear them.

HAIR, HAIR EVERYWHERE

About 1960, males started letting their hair grow, and a lot of people, especially parents, objected. Historically, however, longer hair on men is nothing new. In biblical times, men wore their hair to their shoulders, and in Colonial America longer hair was also fashionable for males of all ages. It really wasn't until the late nineteenth century that men began to wear their hair short. As the years passed, shorter and shorter styles became popular. The crew cut appeared in the 1940s and stayed until the 1950s.

Actually, most boys look better with hair that isn't cropped close to the scalp, but, as with any style, some people go to extremes. Hair flowing halfway to the waist is hard to manage; fortunately, that is an outdated style. Just to the ears or slightly below is the length now preferred by most well-groomed boys and men.

There are still extremes in male hair styles today, of course, but that has more to do with the cut than with the length. Colors that nature never intended and practically shaved heads may be okay if you're a rock star, but they can look silly in a classroom. And they definitely turn prospective employers off! Remember, how you wear your hair makes a statement about the kind of person you are.

Whether you're black or white, Hispanic or Asian; whatever kind of hair you have—curly, wavy or straight, thick or thin—hair is hair and it should be shampooed at least once a week, and more often if it's particularly oily. Every style starts with clean hair. You can shampoo yours when you shower quite easily.

Wet your hair with warm water, step from under the spray and put a dab of shampoo (you don't need much) on your hair. Massage it thoroughly into your hair and scalp. If your hair is really dirty and oily, the first soaping won't give you much lather. Step under the shower and rinse your hair; then apply another dab or two of shampoo and wash your hair again. This time you should see mounds of lather. Rinse out the shampoo completely; your hair will be limp and drab if you leave any in.

Towel-dry and comb your hair. If your hair is very curly or kinky, you'll have an easier time combing it after shampooing if you use a conditioner. After shampooing and rinsing your hair, apply a conditioner. Some conditioners are rinsed out, others are combed through. Then towel your hair dry. You can use a hair dryer to finish the job.

A becoming hair style begins with a proper cut. Today, many barbers are also stylists; they do more than just cut hair. You might like to invest in having a barber-stylist cut your hair. A good one can give you a style that holds its shape and, if your hair is very fine, it can look fuller than it actually is. Very thick hair can be thinned by a stylist.

When deciding how to style your hair, you have to consider the type of hair you have. Straight hair or hair with only a slight natural curl can be worn a little longer than hair that's very thick or curly. This doesn't mean you're stuck with closely cropped hair if yours is thick or curly; it just means you should not let it grow too long.

If you wear an Afro or a square top, remember that the shape and length are important. Like any style, these should be adapted to suit your face size and shape. You want people to see *you*, not merely your hair!

How you part your hair—left side, right side or center—or whether you wear it toward the face or brushed back without a part, can change your appearance for better or for worse. Try different ways to part your hair. Take an honest look at yourself as you part it on the left, on the right and in the center.

[75]

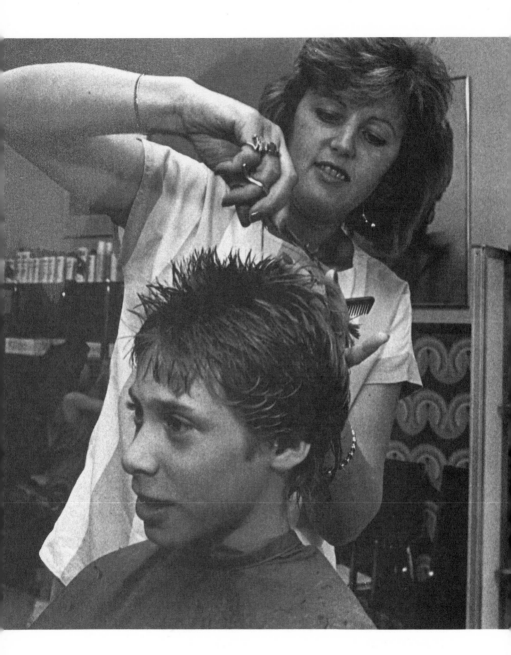

A good haircut makes hair care easier.

If your face is long and narrow, you'll see that a center part makes it look longer and more narrow. If your face is wide, a side part makes it appear wider. Do you have a small face? Then brush your hair back or no one will be able to see what you look like.

Once you've decided which type of part looks best on you, ask Mom and Dad for their opinion. When they discover that you really care about how you look, they might be more willing to go along with the hair style you want.

In order to groom your hair properly, you naturally need the proper tools. A comb and brush and shampoo are essential of course, but you might want to also use conditioners, hair spray, hair dressing or a styling mousse or gel. Your comb should have teeth fine enough to go through the hair from scalp to ends, but not so fine that they break the hair. The brush should have bristles that are firm enough to stimulate the scalp without irritating it.

Both comb and brush should be washed as often as you wash your hair. The easiest way to do this is to soak them in water and detergent for five to ten minutes, then use the comb to get the grime and loose hairs from the brush. The brush can be used to get the dirt from the comb. Then rinse them both completely.

Conditioners, hair sprays, hair dressings and styling mousses or gels are no longer strictly female toiletries. With longer hair, you might find it helpful to use some sort of grooming aid. You

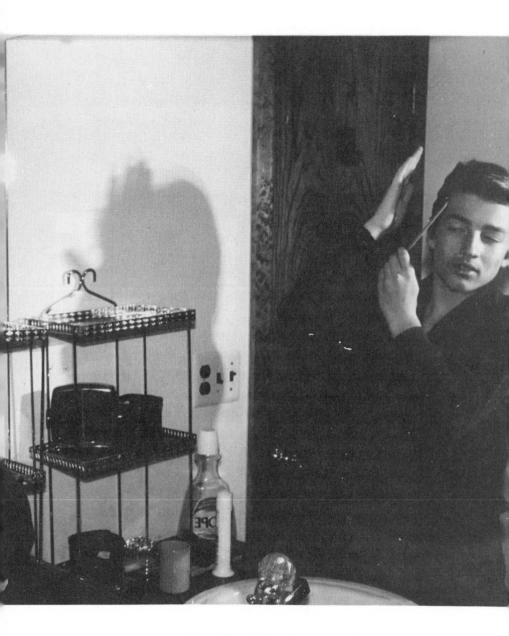

*A comb and brush are
basic hair-grooming tools.*

can choose which one to use by your personal preferences and the requirements of your hair. If you have fine, fly-away hair, a good hair dressing will help to keep it in place. For average hair, experiment with men's hair sprays or styling mousses or gels until you find one that does what you want it to do.

Of course, you don't have to use any of these products. Basically all hair really needs is regular shampooing, combing, brushing and proper cutting when necessary. However, if you decide to use a hair-styling product, be sure to read the directions carefully and to follow them exactly.

When it comes to selecting a shampoo, remember that its main function is to get your hair clean. Therefore, almost any shampoo will do. If you have dandruff, however, use a shampoo formulated to combat that problem. There are also shampoos and conditioners for dry, oily or normal hair. Most conditioners are to be left on the hair for a minute or two, then rinsed out. But a few can be left on the hair; follow the directions on the label for best results.

TEETH, BEARDS, AND OTHER ODDS AND ENDS

There has been a lot printed in newspapers and magazines recently about the decline in cavities. The reason for this is improved dental care, and that begins at home. You need to brush your teeth morning and night and, if possible, after every meal. It's also essential that you see your dentist twice a year.

Practically all toothpastes now contain fluoride to combat cavities; make sure the one you use does, and be sure to use it! Flossing between the teeth with unwaxed dental floss gets out food particles from between your teeth and along the gums. This helps prevent cavities and keeps your gums healthy, so remember to floss after brushing your teeth. In fact, you can carry dental floss with you so that you can use it (in private) when brushing your teeth after a meal isn't practical. But it's a

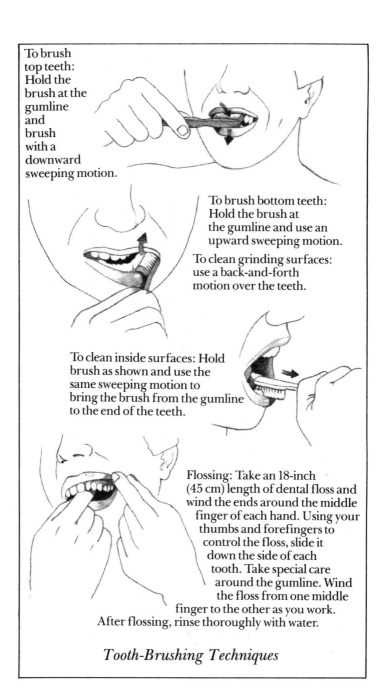

To brush top teeth: Hold the brush at the gumline and brush with a downward sweeping motion.

To brush bottom teeth: Hold the brush at the gumline and use an upward sweeping motion.

To clean grinding surfaces: use a back-and-forth motion over the teeth.

To clean inside surfaces: Hold brush as shown and use the same sweeping motion to bring the brush from the gumline to the end of the teeth.

Flossing: Take an 18-inch (45 cm) length of dental floss and wind the ends around the middle finger of each hand. Using your thumbs and forefingers to control the floss, slide it down the side of each tooth. Take special care around the gumline. Wind the floss from one middle finger to the other as you work. After flossing, rinse thoroughly with water.

Tooth-Brushing Techniques

good idea to keep a toothbrush and toothpaste in your locker at school; the more you brush, the better your teeth will be!

Boys have an additional problem that girls don't; shaving the face. Just about the time that acne pimples may appear, many boys have to start shaving. Using a razor doesn't help get rid of acne, but neither does a beard. Fortunately, few boys have a lot of whiskers in their early teens. If you don't really have to shave yet, you'd be wise to resist the temptation to try Dad's razor for as long as you can.

When you do feel that the fuzz on your face is noticeable, be careful; you don't want to irritate your skin. Use a shaving cream or foam—never use a razor on bare skin. And be sure the blade is sharp; a dull one can cut you instead of the hairs you want to remove. Don't rush when you're shaving; give yourself time so you can do a careful job. And don't shave more often than you actually need to.

Invest in your own razor; they're not expensive nor are razor blades, and you'll avoid arguments with Dad. Electric razors are more expensive, of course, and it would be better to wait until you're older before you buy one. You have to know

Shaving cream or foam
will protect your skin.

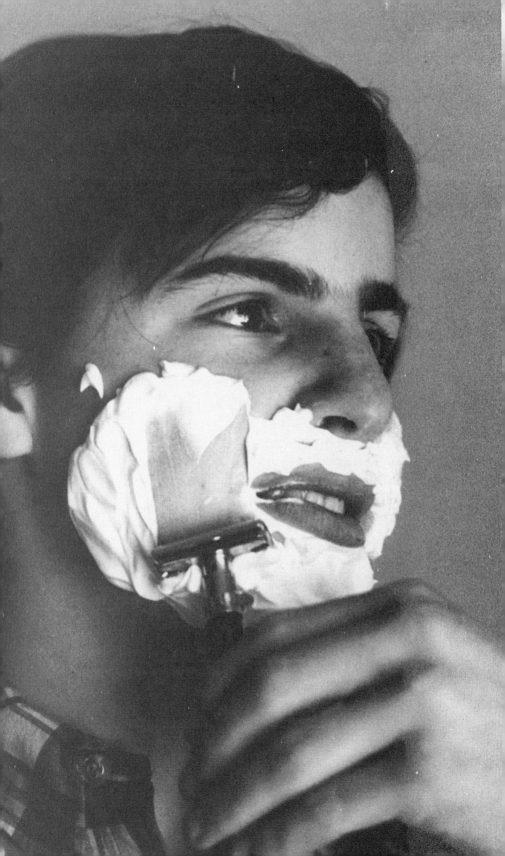

what kind of beard you have—heavy, medium or light—before you can make the right choice; electric razors are not all alike.

Sooner or later, someone will present you with a bottle of cologne. Instead of sprinkling it on the dog or hiding it in the closet, give it a try. There's a wide variety of men's colognes available today, and there is nothing feminine about using them. But it is important to use just a little.

To get an idea of which colognes please you, visit the men's toiletries counter of a department store. There you will find sample bottles so you can try a number of fragrances. Use the inside of your wrist and forearm for testing; don't merely sniff the bottle. Each fragrance develops a different smell on different people. The only way to learn which ones you really like is to dab a little on yourself.

In addition to colognes, men's toiletries also include after-shave lotions that can be used after washing your face. Since practically all of them have an alcohol base, they also help to dry up the excess oil your glands produce at this time.

The language used in some books, movies and even on television may give you the idea that cursing is a way to show you're grown up. Just walking along a street you can hear people using words that are vulgar and obscene. To prove you're just as mature as anybody else, you start cursing, too.

Unfortunately, all that proves is that you're uncouth or stupid or you have a very limited vocabulary—or a combination of all three. Cursing isn't a sign of maturity; it's not manly nor does it impress people favorably. And once you get into the habit of cursing, it's very difficult to break it. Don't fall for the line, "Everybody does it," because everybody *doesn't* curse. Even if most of the kids you know use foul language, you don't have to imitate them.

Many people try to avoid riding buses, subways, and trains when youngsters are going to and from school. If you want to know why, just watch how some of the kids behave; their radios are blaring, they shove and push one another and often innocent bystanders, too.

These kids might not mean to annoy anyone, but they are a nuisance nonetheless. You can do a lot to improve the image of your generation by being more considerate of others when you're in public. If you care enough about yourself to be concerned about your appearance, you should also give some thought to your manners. Good manners are never out of style; use them with your parents, teachers and especially with your friends.

It's considerate of you to use earphones when playing your radio or cassettes, but do you know what listening to music at top volume can do to your hearing? Studies have shown that those whose ears are constantly bombarded by loud sounds—music, jackhammers, jets landing and taking off,

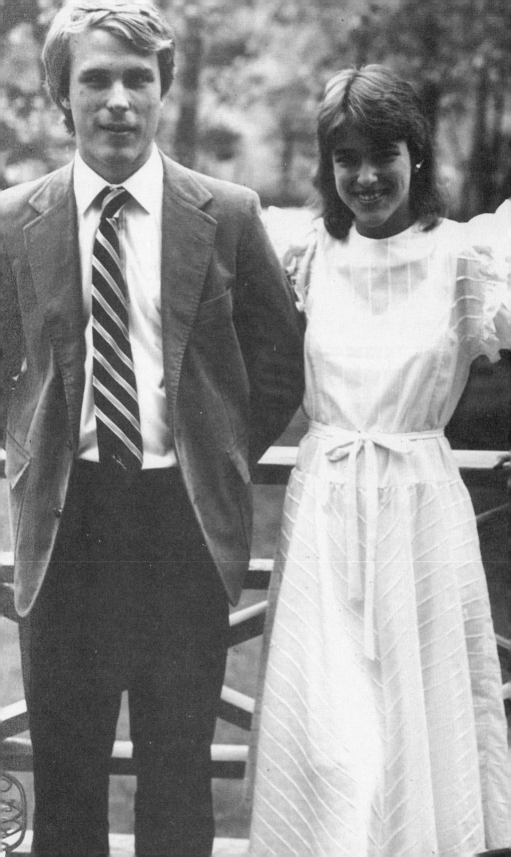

it doesn't matter what—lose a good portion of their hearing. Rock musicians, for example, may find themselves with as much as a 50 percent hearing loss by the time they're thirty. Kids who constantly listen to loud music, with or without earphones, are also in danger of losing some of their hearing. Because the hearing loss is gradual, you might not be immediately aware of it, but if you're not careful you may have to exchange those earphones for a hearing aid in the future.

What does all this have to do with good grooming? It's simple: good grooming is not only a matter of how you look, but how you act. The best-dressed boy in the world can still lack friends if he's loud and uncouth. And you know the good impression you make when you're reasonably polite to everyone with whom you come into contact. When good grooming and good manners become second nature to you, you can face the world with confidence.

*Good grooming helps
you feel ready to face
the world.*

———————♂———————

GOOD
GROOMING
CHECKLIST

Here's a list of things you should remember about grooming.

It will help you keep tabs on yourself to make sure you haven't overlooked anything.

- ☐ Remember to scrub your nails when you shower.
- ☐ Shampoo your hair at least once a week; more often if it's oily.
- ☐ Check your deodorant; is it time to buy another?
- ☐ Wash your face thoroughly at least twice a day. Keep your hands away from it except when washing it or applying medication.
- ☐ Brush your teeth morning and at bedtime as well as after every meal.
- ☐ Wear clean underwear and socks every day.

□ Take clothes to the cleaner when necessary; soiled washable clothes belong in the hamper.
□ Eat smart whether you want to lose or gain weight and even if your weight isn't a problem.
□ Get enough sleep every night.
□ Walk tall and proud and exercise every day.

For Further Reading

To learn more about the subjects covered in *Good Grooming for Boys*, look for these books in your school or public library:

Abrams, Joy, Ruth Richards and Pam Gray. *Look Good, Feel Good: Through Yoga, Grooming, Nutrition.* New York: Holt Rinehart & Winston, 1978.

Arnold, Caroline. *Too Fat? Too Thin? Do You Have a Choice?* New York: Morrow, 1984.

Eagles, Douglas. *Your Weight.* New York: Franklin Watts, 1982.

Englebardt, Stanley L. *How to Get in Shape for Sports.* New York: Lothrop, Lee and Shepard, 1976.

Gilbert, Sara. *Fat Free: Common Sense for Young Weight Worriers.* New York: Macmillan, 1975.

————. *You Are What You Eat.* New York: Macmillan, 1977.

Jacobs, Karen. *Health.* Chicago: Children's Press, 1981.

Kiss, Michaeline. *Yoga for Young People.* Indianapolis: Bobbs-Merrill, 1971.

LeMaster, Leslie Jean. *Nutrition.* Chicago: Children's Press, 1985.

Lewis, Nancy. *Keeping in Shape.* New York: Franklin Watts, 1976.

Neff, Fred. *Keeping Fit.* Minneapolis: Lerner Publications, 1977.

Novick, Nelson Lee, M.D. *Skin Care for Teens.* New York: Franklin Watts, 1988.

Peavy, Linda, and Ursula Smith. *Food, Nutrition and You.* New York: Scribners, 1982.

Index

[93]

About the Author

Rubie Saunders has been deeply involved in the writing and editing of books and magazines for young readers all of her professional life.

She has written more than one hundred and fifty articles and a dozen books, including *The Concise Guide to Baby Sitting*.

A graduate of Hunter College in New York City, she was elected to the Hunter Hall of Fame. She enjoys working with youngsters and has received a distinguished service award from Cub Scout Pack 371 in Brooklyn.

She now lives in New Rochelle, New York, where she serves on the Board of Education.